The Ultimate Mediterranean Diet Cookbook for Beginners

Lose Weight Rapidly and Never Let It Back, Rebuild Your Body and Be Confident Again, Enjoy a Easy Comfortable Lifestyle

By Linda C. Green

Table of Contents

Chapter 6: Amazing Mediterranean Diet Snacks........................... 59

Chapter 7: Great Mediterranean Diet Desserts..................67

The Final Words..80

Preface

If you are looking for an effective and actionable way of losing your excess weight;
If you want to have a healthy lifestyle just as others;
If you want to eat what you want or like, meantime live happy without illness;
Then please keep reading, you will find answers by following this book.

This book is all about Mediterranean Diet living. It is the most comprehensive and easy-to-follow guide for beginners and advanced users. Too many people have got their dream body weight and prevented disease from them. You are a lucky dog, as you really have chosen the right book for you and your family or friends around you!

This Mediterranean Diet cookbook is an ultimate guide, with simple-to-prepare delicious recipes to lead you to a successful Mediterranean diet. By following it, you will know all essentials about Mediterranean Diet in a short. Such as:
The history of the Mediterranean Diet
Science Reasons behind the Mediterranean Diet
Great Advantages of Following the Mediterranean Diet
Actionable Weight Loss Tips about Mediterranean Diet
Many Effective Tips to a Successful Mediterranean Diet
What Foods to Eat or Avoid
Some Useful Advice on Eating Out
More and more...

In this book, the wide variety of food choices might surprise you, and you will not go hungry. Recipes for some healthy snacks are also included to help the adjustment. This is not a diet of calorie counting, but rather a diet that eliminates unhealthy foods. It is a diet whereby you CAN lose weight, by eating the healthy Ingredients mentioned in this book. Make sure you have smaller portion sizes if you wish to lose weight. Moreover, always include essential daily exercise, to keep a healthy heart.

After finish reading the first chapter about Mediterranean Diet, you will dive into the recipe chapters.All recipes are easy to follow and categorized into common types: **Breakfasts, Lunches, Dinners, Snacks, Desserts**.

Now let's start to discover some interesting facts, then prepare tasty healthy recipes for our Mediterranean journey. Wish you a happy and successful Mediterranean Diet living!

Chapter 1: Essential Knowledge of the Mediterranean Diet

What's the Mediterranean Diet?

It's a specific diet by removing processed foods and/ or high in saturated fats. It's not only effective about losing weight, but also regard as a very healthy lifestyle. It is about ingesting traditional Ingredients consumed by those who live in the Mediterranean basin for a long time. Their diets never changed, so they must be doing something right. This is a diet rich in fruits, vegetables, and fish. Cooking with olive oil is a fundamental ingredient and is an ideal replacement for saturated fats and trans fats. Vegetables and fruits grow well in the heat of the Mediterranean continents, so it's not surprising that the locals devour plenty of them. Studies show that the people who live in these regions live longer and better lives. Changing your own eating habits to one that is proven to be healthy is a good enough reason to begin.

History of the Mediterranean Diet

Mediterranean cuisine refers to food types eaten in countries that lay within the regions of the Mediterranean basin. There are around 22 countries situated in the Mediterranean basin, notably: Italy, Greece and Southern France, all bringing a wide cultural diversity to the menu. There are also foods from Eastern Europe, and the added touches from the Eastern shores of the African continent. There is no single diet, as it is an accumulation of regional variances. This lends an eclectic variety of Ingredients, and various ways of cooking them. The influence of the Mediterranean diet began to spread throughout the world in the 1950's. The hot climate has a major influence on the diet. With little rainfall, there is little grazing for cattle. That is the reason the indigenous people of these lands turn to what they can cultivate. The sun provides them with an abundance of rich fruits and various vegetables. Seafood also plays a major role in meals on the coastlines of the Mediterranean Sea. Hardy animals that are able to survive dry conditions, such as goats and chickens add to the cuisine as well.

Science Reasons behind the Mediterranean Diet

The ever-growing problem of cardiovascular disease is a major trouble of the modern Western diet, which increased in the 20th century. In the 1970s has been connected to the Western dietary intake of high carb and sugary foods. This led scientists to wonder why those living in the Mediterranean regions have such low rates of this deadly condition. The main study in the 1980's was known as the MONICA (Multinational Monitoring of trends and determinants in Cardiovascular disease). It collated over 10 years' worth of data, and included 21countries. The results were so pivotal, that they are the foundation of the belief that this is the best diet on the planet. Another study in 2003, took 772 participants, and the tests lasted 3 months. Again, the results showed a larger DECREASE in blood sugar and blood pressure levels, for those on the Mediterranean style diet, than for those on a low-fat diet. In other studies, the increased consumption of nuts (over a 5year period) has shown a 16-63% REDUCED risk of cardiovascular death. The low mortality rate of those who cook daily with olive oil, is just one of the many excellent reasons to change to the Mediterranean way of eating.

Great Advantages of Following the Mediterranean Diet

With the findings of a 30% reduction in heart disease, published in 2013 from a study by the New England Journal of Medicine called PREDIMED we should take these constant studies seriously. Isn't that inviting enough to encourage you to change your diet? How about the studies that proved Mediterranean foods stop the brain shrinking with age, which has been correlated to the high intake of plant based foods?

The food on the tables of the Mediterranean basin families are without a doubt more wholesome and nutritious than the typical Western diet. The Ingredients include fish (at least twice a week), providing high protein along with omega3 fat. Whilst on the topic of fats; the olive oil they use comes from the olives they personally cultivate. Olive oil is full of monounsaturated fatty acids. These are good fats with many benefits. One is that it helps reduce the risk of heart disease and strokes. Other foods are outsized portions of vegetables and fruit, nuts, seeds, legumes and basically any whole grains.

What you will NOT find on their tables are the high in saturated fats, sugars and salt processed foods. These foods contribute to the development of cardiovascular disease in the Western diet.

Is It Really Good for Weight Loss?

What does it mean then, to change your eating habits to integrate Mediterranean foods? One thing for sure, you can lose weight and still have a variety of Ingredients in your meals. With around 20 different countries influencing the diet, it's guaranteed you will find plenty of options for healthily eating. There are no strict rules, just stick to the Mediterranean influence and it will help you shed those pounds. There is plenty of protein if you follow the diet, which will give you the satiated effect. Not only that, most of it makes your body healthier; no excess fats build up and sent to store. Moreover, because you feel healthier, it encourages you to exercise more. Whilst work outs do not necessarily help in losing weight, they help in many other ways. As your blood pumps around faster, your heart can cope better. Muscles and bones become stronger. The more endorphins you produce in exercise, the better your mood. Therefore, it is not just about food, it about feeling good and WANTING to be healthier.

Menu options aren't difficult, even when you eat out. Choose a Mediterranean influenced meal with fish or poultry, and cooked in olive oil. Pile on the vegetables and fruit along with it. Indulge in pastas and pizzas, but in small portions.

What Will be Happened While Following the Mediterranean Diet?

Not only your heart that will thank you for the consumption of a Mediterranean style diet, there are other changes that will happen to your body:
- Lower blood sugar levels. Ideal for Diabetes Type II.
- Strengthen muscles and bones. Studies have shown a 70% increase in strength for the elderly on a Mediterranean Diet.
- Eating healthy antioxidants reduces the effects of brain shrinkage in old age. This in turn will reduce the risk of neuro-degeneration diseases, such as Parkinson's and Alzheimer's.
- Reduce the risk of cancerous cells developing.
- Increase energy and better concentrations skills.
- Reduce chances of neurological diseases.
- Helps fight inflammations.
- Produce higher rates of dopamine in the brain, leading to a feeling of well-being and improved mood.
- All that vitamin E will improve skin condition and glow.
- Lose weight, so long as you monitor portion sizes and exercise regularly.

Lose Weight Fast During the Mediterranean Diet

When you think of pizzas and pastas, you do not associate these foods with weight loss. Whilst you can still eat carbs on this diet, you will not eat large portions of them. Pasta tends to be a side dish, about a half of a cup, set on a great plate of vegetables and salad.
- The focus on how Mediterranean people eat, is not just about the food; it includes such things as smaller portions and exercising. Also, their pace of life is less demanding.
- Feel fuller for longer, as you will be eating more protein-based Ingredients. This will deter you from eating snacks between meals. However, some relevant snack recipes are included.
- The Ingredients of the Mediterranean style diet naturally tend to be low in calories and high in fiber. This is the perfect combination to rid the excess fat reserves.

- Go for the low-fat options such as Greek yogurt, milk and cheese when choosing dairy products.
- Red meat should be consumed only a couple of times a month, if at all. White meats are fine, so long they are the lean options.
- The secret of this way of eating is the olive oil. Use nothing else but extra virgin olive oil (EVOO) and you too will live a long and slim life.

Some Effective Tips to a Successful Mediterranean Diet

If you can maintain a healthy Mediterranean Diet, the list of health benefits is endless.

- Eating healthier can lead to a longer life. Not only does it increase your lifespan, but also makes you feel healthier and fitter for longer; well into your golden age.
- This is not a restrictive diet. With our recipes, you will learn that you are eliminating certain types of food from your diet. Yet, with so many remaining, you can enjoy cooking and eating with delight.
- A Mediterranean style diet is not expensive, after all, it's up to you how much to spend on food and where to buy it. It's pricier to order take outs or to frequent meals at restaurants, so try to limit them.
- You can also go vegetarian and bulk up your meals with legumes, as opposed to having meats. They not only provide ample protein, but also a great amount of fiber.
- As we have said before, and will continue to reiterate, the secret is in the oil. ALWAYS use olive oil. Buy the best you can and if you can afford it, get the EVOO. If you need oil that gets hot without smoking, use light olive oil. Your heart will be grateful for the rest of your life.

Should I Take Exercise During the Mediterranean Diet?

Anyone looking to lose weight should ensure they exercise every day, no matter what their dietary intake is. This does not mean to dash off to a sports club and pay expensive fees. A healthy brisk walk at least twice a week (of at least 6000 feet), takes about an hour. Or 4 x 30 minute energetic exercises, such as walking, swimming, or invent a home workout. That is the minimum guideline. How much extra exercise you do on top of that depends on how much time you want to spare. Exercise alone does not mean you will lose weight. What you can do though, is increase your daily calories by about an extra 200 (if you're on a minimum or around 1600 calories), on days when you exercise. Already you are doing your heart a great favor by being on a heart-friendly diet. Combine that with the basic exercise and you will have more energy and a healthier body. The Mediterranean Diet, combined with exercise, will help toward losing weight and keep you healthy.

What Foods Should We Eat?

Replacing saturated and hydrogenated fats with olive oil is one of the major differences in the Mediterranean diet. Everything is cooked in olive oil. That includes salad dressings and marinades. Of course, they grow their own olives in the Mediterranean regions, so it's no surprise this oil is so popular. Other healthy choices include olives and avocados. Primarily, you are increasing your plant-based foods. Don't cook with butter when a recipe asks to use olive oil. Don't use sugar to make foods tasty, use herbs and spices instead. Red meat does not have to be off the menu (prepare only a couple of times every month), but white lean meat is better. Fish is also an important ingredient in this diet, and served at least twice a week.

This quick guide gives an idea of the major foodstuffs. Think of it as a pyramid, with the top Ingredients of the list making the large foundation. As you go down the list, the pyramid gets smaller, so eat less of these Ingredients:

1. The foundation of the pyramid consists of being substantial and social. Having family meals, dancing with friends, walking, and sports. These are all activities that people who live in hot climates always do, but all of it plays a role in the Mediterranean way of life.

2. All vegetables, even including tubers (root vegetables. Fruits- from the apple to the sweet fig; dates, grapes, melons, strawberries, bananas, kiwis. Legumes- including peas, lentils, peanuts, chickpeas and other types of beans. Whole grains- such as oats, rice (wild or brown are better), rye, barley, buckwheat, corn, pasta (whole wheat better), whole-wheat bread (not buttered). Nuts- for example hazelnut, cashew, walnut, almond (but

only a handful daily). Seeds- like the sunflower and pumpkin. Herbs and spices a plenty, with garlic and basil, nutmeg and cinnamon being the favorites. Also, drink plenty of water.

3. Seafood and oily fish, from salmon to sardines, shrimp to oyster.
4. Poultry, but mostly chicken and duck. Dairy such as Greek yogurt, cheese and milk. Eggs. Red wine (no more than 5oz daily - if you miss a day, no doing a double). If you don't like alcohol, then drink purple grape juice.
5. Other meats and sweet things are consumed in small amounts.

What Foods to Avoid?

When learning any new diet, it's also important to learn which foods should NOT be included. Another important factor is to read the labels on everything. It is the only way to be completely aware of what goes into the food you eat. Here's a quick guide for inspiration:

Foods considered as processed, such as sausages and bread should be eaten in moderation. DON'T have any that are super processed, such as hotdogs, take outs, pastries. They are exceptionally high in sugars and salt, Ingredients and proven to be linked to cancer risks.

Check the sugar levels if they are labeled as "low fat"

STOP adding sugar to your tea and coffee.

ALWAYS check that sugar content is not high on the Ingredients list. The higher it is on the list, the more there is in the food contents. Many readymade foods such as sauces, milk and even bread have it.

AVOID foods made with refined grains. That means that the process has removed all the important dietary fiber, such as white bread, white flour, white rice, white pasta etc.

AVOID bad fats and refined oils. Anything labeled with *trans fats* or *hydrogenated fats* is bad for you. These can be in foods such as margarines, cakes, even microwave popcorn. Don't use oils such as canola, soy, soybean etc. outlearn about the types of fats used in the food you eat, whenever you can. DO NOT buy if "trans fats" is on the label. Take outs will not have labels, but they use lots of trans fats for cooking. BEWARE of them.

Any Useful Advice on Eating Out?

Just because you enjoy eating at restaurants, does not mean you have to ditch the diet. The Mediterranean way of eating positively encourages making meals a social event. It can be a time to get together and unwind. Their way of life might be slower, but there is no reason why you cannot incorporate it into your own new lifestyle. Here are a few tips to help you when eating out:

- As you take a seat, have a glass of water. Studies have shown that drinking 17ounces of water prior to a meal, gives you 44% chance not to overeat, therefore assists in weight loss.
- Avoid breadbaskets. Eat whole-wheat bread at best, but save that for home and in moderation.
- Avoid fried foods, unless you are confident they are cooked in olive oil. The only to find is to ask, if you're bold enough.
- Skip the appetizer, or share one at the very least.
- For your main course, chose chicken, or lean pork if you prefer a meat dish. Or consider having fish instead. Better yet, have a vegetarian plate
- Avoid dishes with sauces. Chances are, they have ample sugar and salt to make them palatable. Again, you could ask, but if you are at a chain restaurant, they may not even know the answer as it comes ready made in bulk. That's not a nice reflection!
- Choose plenty of vegetables, even order more as a side dish.
- Avoid salad dressings.
- Fruit for dessert is always better. If you can't resist a pudding; share it with a few friends, this way you only have a couple of spoons.
- Enjoy one glass of red wine, and then drink water for the rest of the meal.
- Chew slowly until all the food is masticated, and easy to swallow.
- Think about the flavors of your food as you chew. Simply said, don't just eat by design- discover the flavors within.
- Sit down and enjoy the food. Appreciate what you taste and consume
- Restaurant portions may be large, so get into the habit of leaving some food on your plate.

Chapter 2: Mouth-watering Mediterranean Diet Breakfast

Scrambled Eggs and Spinach

Serves: 1
Preparation Time: 15 minutes
Ingredients
2 eggs
1 tsp butter
1 cup spinach leaves, shredded

2 baby plum tomatoes, chopped
Salt and pepper to taste

Instructions
- Heat the butter in a small pan. Add the spinach and tomatoes, until spinach has wilted.
- Whisk eggs and pour egg mixture into the pan with spinach and tomatoes. Scramble the mix with a fork. Once cooked through, season with salt and pepper and serve immediately.

Eggs and Avocado on Toast

Serves: 1
Preparation Time: 15 minutes
Ingredients
1 egg
1 slice whole meal bread
1/2 avocado, peeled and thinly sliced
Salt and pepper to taste
Instructions
- In a small pan, boil the egg until medium soft (apx 8 mins).
- Toast the bread, and while still warm, lay the avocado slices on it. Use a knife to spread the avocado.
- When the egg is ready, remove the shell and cut into quarters. Place on top of the avocado. Add salt and pepper.

Spinach and Tomato Frittata

Serves: 2
Preparation Time: 15 minutes
Ingredients

6 eggs
1/2 cup skim milk
3 baby plum tomatoes, diced
1/2 cup Greek olives, halved and pitted

1 cup spinach leaves, chopped
1 tbsp feta, roughly crumbled
1 tsp dried oregano
1 tbsp extra virgin olive oil
Salt and pepper to taste

Instructions

- Preheat oven to 400F
- Lightly whisk the eggs. Add remaining Ingredients and mix. Add salt and pepper. Grease an 8in flan dish and add the mixture. Bake for 20 mins or until eggs are set. Cut into wedges and serve hot or cold.

Greek Mashed Fava Beans

Serves: 2
Ingredients

16 oz can fava beans, rinsed and drained
1 slice whole-wheat bread
1/2 onion, finely chopped
2 cloves garlic minced

Preparation Time: 20 minutes

1 tsp cumin
2 lemons, juiced
1/2 cup water
1 tbsp extra virgin olive oil
Salt and pepper to taste

Instructions

- Heat the oil in a pan and sauté onions for 2 mins. Add garlic and cumin and cook for another minute. Add the fava beans and water. Bring to a boil, then reduce heat, cover and cook for 10 mins. Remove lid and continue cooking until most of the liquid reduced.
- Pour the mixture into a mixing bowl and add the lemon juice. Crush the mixture into a chunky consistency with a potato masher.
- Serve with warm pita bread. For variety and a more substantial meal, top it with two hard-boiled eggs, quartered.

Mediterranean Fruit Salad

Serves: 2
Preparation Time: 15 minutes
Ingredients

3 persimmons, NOT soft ones
12oz grapes, cut in half
1 tbsp lemon juice

8 mint leaves very finely sliced
14oz sliced toasted almonds
Honey to taste.

Instructions

Peel the persimmons then cut into wedges. In a bowl, combine with all other Ingredients and stir well.
Nutritional Value Per serving: Calories 159, Fat 4g (Sat 0g), Carbs32g, Fiber 5g, Protein 3g

Eggs and Salad Pita

Serves: 2
Preparation Time: 20 minutes
Ingredients

4 eggs, hard boiled
2 whole-wheat pita bread, halved.
1/2 cup of hummus. (recipe in Snacks)

1/2 cucumber, thinly sliced
2 tomatoes roughly chopped
Fresh ground black pepper to taste

Instructions

Bring water to a boil and add the eggs, boil for approximately 7-8 minutes for hard-boiled. Warm the pita and with a sharp knife cut open pockets at the edge. Slice the eggs and sprinkle with pepper. Divide the hummus between the pitas and spread into the pocket. Add the egg slices, the tomatoes and cucumber.

Sardine and Egg Artichoke

Serves: 2

Preparation Time: 10 minutes

Ingredients

4oz can sardines in tomato sauce

5 tbsp canned artichoke hearts, chopped

2 eggs

1 cup green lettuce, shredded

Salt and pepper to taste

Instructions

In a small bowl add sardines and artichokes, and mash into a lumpy paste. In a small oven dish, spread the sardine mix and break 2 eggs on top, careful not to burst the yokes. Sprinkle with salt and pepper and bake in oven for 10 mins. Serve on top of green lettuce.

Lemon Scone

Servings: 12

Preparation Time: 20 minutes

Ingredients

7 oz all purpose flour, (or half with whole wheat flour)

3oz butter

2 tbsp sugar

2 tsp baking soda

3 fl oz cup buttermilk

2 tsp lemon juice

1/2 tsp salt

Frosting

1 cup powdered sugar

1-2 tsp lemon juice

Instructions

- Preheat oven to 400F
- In a large bowl, combine flour, baking soda, sugar and salt, and mix. Cut butter into small pieces, and with clean hands or in a pastry blender rub into the flour mix. It should resemble breadcrumbs. The lesser the handling- the better. Add lemon juice and buttermilk. Shape the dough into a ball and then flatten out on a floured surface to get the thickness you want. Cut into 12 even pieces. Place the scones onto a baking tray and bake for 12 mins.
- In a smaller bowl, add the powdered sugar and lemon juice, and mix until combined. Once the scones are done, drizzle this over them.

Nutritional Value per serving: Calories 175, Fat 4g (of which sat 3g); Carbs 3g, Fiber 1g, Protein 3g.

Zucchini Frittata

Servings: 4
Preparation Time: 25 minutes
Ingredients

2 zucchinis, sliced into rounds of 1/4 inch thick
2 oz goat cheese, crumbled
8 eggs

1 clove garlic, minced
2 tbsp milk
1 tbsp extra virgin olive oil
Salt and pepper to taste

Instructions

- Heat the oil in a skillet, and sauté the zucchini and garlic for around 5 mins.
- In a large bowl, whisk the eggs and milk, adding salt and pepper. Stir into the zucchini mix. Top with cheese and bake for 10 mins.
- Leave to stand for 3 mins when firm; it should come out of the pan easier when cooled off.
- Cut into 4 wedges.

Nutritional Values per serving: Calories 134, Fat 8g (Sat 3g), Carbs 3g, Fiber 1g, Protein 12g.

Yogurt and Figs

Servings: 4
Preparation Time: 15 minutes
Ingredients

8 oz fresh figs, halved
1/4 cup pistachios, finely chopped2 cups Greek yogurt
2 tbsp honey
1 tsp ground cinnamon

Instructions

- In a skillet, heat 1 tbsp honey and place figs cut side down to cook for 5 mins.
- Serve with yogurt, sprinkled with cinnamon and nuts. Drizzle the remaining honey over the top.

Honey Yogurt and Melon

Servings: 8
Preparation Time: 10 minutes
Ingredients
1 honeydew melon, cut into 16 wedges
3 cups plain Greek yogurt
1/2 cup fresh mint leaves, chopped
1/4 cup honey
Instructions
- Place melon on a platter.
- Pour yogurt into a bowl, drizzle with honey then garnish with mint.

Nutty Oats and Apple

Servings: 1
Preparation Time: 10 minutes
Ingredients
1/4 cup of quick cooking oats
2 tbsp walnuts, chopped
1 tsp flax seed
3 tbsp honey
1/2 cup skim milk
Half of an apple, peeled and sliced
Instructions
In a microwave-safe bowl, combine ALL Ingredients, and cook on high for 1 min. Remove and stir. Cook for another minute. Let stand for 1 min before serving.

Granola

Servings: 7

Preparation Time: 10 minutes

Ingredients

5 cups of rolled oats

1 cup coconut, shredded

1 cup almond slivers

1/4 cup honey

3 tbsp extra virgin olive oil

Instructions

- Set the oven to 250F
- In a large bowl, combine the oats, almonds, shredded coconut and mix well. Add the oil and honey. Spread a thin layer over 2 flat oven trays, and bake for 90 minutes. Remove and stir every 20 mins. Allow to cool, before breaking up and storing in a sealed container.

Whole-wheat Pancakes

Servings: 6

Preparation Time: 15 minutes

Ingredients

1 cup of rolled oats

2 cups plain Greek yogurt

2 large eggs

1/2 cup whole-wheat flour

1 tsp baking soda

1 tbsp flax seed

2 tbsp honey

2 tbsp extra virgin olive oil

Instructions

- Mix the oats, flour, baking soda and flax seed in a large bowl. Add yogurt, eggs, 1 tbsp oil and whisk until smooth. Let it rest for at least 20 mins (put in the fridge if longer).
- In a frying pan heat 1 tsp oil, and pour 1/4 cup of batter. Keep adding more oil if needed. Cook until it begins to firm, then flip and cook other side until brown, approx. 2 mins each side.
- Serve warm with yogurt and honey drizzled over. You can also include pieces of fruit.

Cheesy Bacon Oatmeal

Servings: 4

Preparation Time: 15 minutes

Ingredients

8 slices of bacon

1/2 cup of rolled oats

2 cups whole milk

1/4 cup water

1 large tomato, sliced

1/2 cup mild shredded cheese

1 tsp honey

Instructions

- Cook bacon until crispy. Set aside to cool then crumble.
- In a large pan, bring milk and water to boil. Add oats and simmer for 25 mins, stirring occasionally. Stir in cheese and honey. Serve in 4 bowls and sprinkle with crispy bacon pieces.

Chapter 4: Graceful Mediterranean Diet Lunches

Avocado and Tomato Salad

Serves: 4
Preparation Time: 20 minutes
Ingredients
- 1 avocado peeled and roughly chopped
- 1 cucumber peeled and sliced
- 10oz cherry tomatoes, quartered
- Small red onion, diced
- 4oz feta cheese, crumbled
- 3.5 oz olives of choice, halved and pitted
- 2 sprigs flat leaf parsley, chopped

Dressing:
- 2 tbsp extra virgin olive oil
- 2 tbsp red wine vinegar
- 1 clove garlic, finely minced
- 1/4 tsp dried oregano
- 1/4 tsp sugar
- Salt and pepper to taste

Instructions
- For the dressing, add all the Ingredients in a jar with a lid. Shake until it emulsifies.
- For the salad, mix the avocado, tomatoes, olives, cucumber, onion, parsley in a bowl.
- Pour the dressing over the salad, and toss until all Ingredients are covered.
- Top the salad with cheese. Best when marinating in cool temperature for 10 minutes.

Chickpea and Pepper Salad

Serves: 4
Preparation Time: 30 minutes
Ingredients
- 1 1/2 cups chick peas, washed and drained
- 2 cups cherry tomatoes, halved
- 1 cucumber, deseeded and diced
- 1 red bell pepper, diced
- 1 small red onion, diced
- 1/2 cup olives of choice, halved and pitted
- 1 cup feta cheese crumbled into large chunks

Dressing:
- 2 tbsp extra virgin olive oil
- 1/4 cup lemon juice
- 1/4 tsp dried oregano
- 1/2 cup fresh parsley, chopped
- Salt and pepper to taste

Instructions
- For the dressing, add all the Ingredients into a lidded jar. Shake until it emulsifies.
- For the salad, add the Ingredients into a large bowl and mix.
- Pour the dressing onto salad, and toss.
- Best left to stand in cool temperature for 10 minutes, so it can marinade.

Chicken and Couscous Burrito

Serves: 4
Preparation Time: 30 minutes
Ingredients
1/3 cup whole-wheat couscous
1lb chicken breast, cut into large cubes
1 medium salad tomato, chopped
1 cup cucumber, skinned and chopped
1 tsp ready prepared minced garlic
1/4 cup fresh mint, chopped
1 cup fresh parsley leaves, chopped
1/4 cup lemon juice
2 tbsp extra virgin olive oil
Salt and pepper to taste
Four 10' tomato or spinach tortilla wraps
Instructions
- In a small pan, cover the couscous with boiling water. Cover and set aside for 5 mins.
- In a medium sized bowl, add the parsley, mint, lemon juice, oil, garlic, salt and pepper and whisk together. Place chicken pieces in another bowl and coat with 1 tbsp of mint mix. Cook chicken on a skillet for 3-5 minutes both sides.
- Fluff up the couscous with a fork and add the remaining mint mixture, tomato, and cucumber.
- Spoon 3/4 cup of couscous on each wrap. Divide the cooked chicken between them. Roll up, tucking the ends inside first. Cut in half to serve.

Nutritional Value: per wrap: Calories 510, Carbs 55g, Fats 18g, Fiber 6g, Protein 32g

Buffet Bento

Serves: 1
Preparation Time: 30 minutes
Ingredients
1/4 cup canned chickpeas, rinsed and drained
3oz chicken breast, cooked and cubed
1/4 cup cucumber, diced
1/4 cup cherry tomatoes, halved
1 cup grapes
1 cup olives of choice, halved and pitted
2 tbsp hummus
1 oz feta cheese, crumbled
1 whole-wheat pita bread, quartered
1 tbsp fresh parsley leaves, chopped
1/2 tsp extra virgin olive oil
1 tsp red wine vinegar
Black pepper to taste
Instructions
- In a medium bowl, combine cucumber, tomatoes, feta, parsley, olives, vinegar and black pepper. Whisk together. Place in a medium container with a lid.
- Store the hummus, chicken, grapes and pita in their own containers with covers.
- When you are ready to eat your single-serving buffet, open all the containers.

Nutritional Value: Calories 495, Carbs 60g, Fats 14g, Fiber 8g, Protein 35g

Whole-wheat Cheese and Avocado Sandwich

Serves: 1

Preparation Time: 20 minutes

Ingredients

2 slices whole-wheat bread
1/4 cup parmesan cheese, grated
1/4 cup avocado, peeled, pitted, and mashed
1 medium tomato, sliced
1 cup lettuce and spinach, shredded
2 tsp balsamic vinegar
1 pear, quartered

Instructions

- Spread the avocado on one slice of bread. Sprinkle cheese,, then top with tomatoes.
- Place both pieces of bread under a hot grill. Remove the bare slice once browned the other when the cheese melts.
- Add the greens, and drizzle with balsamic vinegar. Place the other toasted slice of bread on top and gently press together.
- Cut in half and serve on a plate with the pear.

Nutritional Value: Calories 440, Carbs 63g, Fats 15g (which 5g saturated), Fiber 14g, Protein 18g.

Feta and Couscous Wrap

Serves: 4
Preparation Time: 15 minutes
Ingredients
1/2 cup whole-wheat couscous.
1 cup of feta cheese, crumbled
2 garlic cloves, minced
2 red bell peppers, finely sliced
1 tomato, diced
1 cucumber, diced
4 sun-dried tomato wraps
1/2 cup boiling water
2 tbsp lemon juice
2 tbsp extra virgin olive oil
Salt and pepper to taste
Instructions
- Boil water in a pan. Remove from heat and add the couscous to water, stir and cover. Let stand for 5 minutes.
- To make the dressing, combine garlic, mint, salt, pepper, lemon juice, and olive oil into a small bowl, and mix well. Stir in the feta, couscous, cucumber and chopped tomato. Divide the couscous mixture evenly between the four wraps. Roll up, folding the ends first.
- Serve with a simple green salad, sprinkled with olive oil.

Creamy Chicken Pita

Serves: 2
Preparation Time: 15 minutes
Ingredients
2 pieces whole-wheat pitas
1 chicken breast, skinned and cut into chunks
1 medium tomato, diced
1 crushed garlic clove
1/2 cucumber, small cubes
1/2 tsp dried oregano
1 tbsp EVOO
Marinade:
1/2 cup plain Greek yogurt
1 tsp dried oregano
1 tbsp EVOO
Salt and pepper to taste
Greek Sauce:
2 tbsp mayonnaise
1 tbsp milk
1 tbsp white wine vinegar
1/2 tsp lemon juice
1/4 tsp sugar
Pinch garlic powder
Salt and pepper to taste
Instructions
- In a medium bowl, whisk together yogurt, 1 tbsp of oil, 1 tsp dried oregano, salt and pepper. Add the chicken and stir until thoroughly coated. Marinade in fridge for minimum of 2hrs, ideally overnight.
- Greek Sauce: Mix all **Ingredients** together and store in fridge
- Remove chicken from marinade. Heat 1 tbsp oil in skillet and broil the chicken over a high heat. Add garlic, oregano and cook for around 6 mins, tossing chicken on all sides.
- Once cooked, place chicken into the Greek sauce. Divide equally between the pita bread; either on top, or stuffed. Add tomatoes and cucumber.

Hummus and Chickpea Pita

Serves: 1
Preparation Time: 15 minutes
Ingredients
1 whole-wheat pita bread, cut in half
1/4 cup hummus (recipe ch6)
1/4 cup chickpeas, rinsed and drained
2 tbsp feta cheese, crumbled
2 tsp sun-dried tomatoes
1/4 cup carrots, shredded
Handful baby spinach, rinsed and drained
2 tsp olives of choice, chopped and pitted
1 tbsp EVOO
Salt and pepper to taste
Instructions
- Warm the pita, and cut the top of the pocket open with a knife. Distribute the hummus, chickpeas, carrots, tomatoes, spinach and olives into each pocket. Drizzle the oil inside and top with feta and salt and pepper.
- May be refrigerated for up to 4 hours.

Spinach Orzo Soup

Serves: 6

Preparation Time: 20 minutes

Ingredients

1 cup long grain rice
4 eggs
1 white onion, finely diced
10 oz frozen spinach, thawed and drained
4 garlic cloves, minced
3 lemons, juiced
1 tsp red pepper flakes
3 tsp fresh parsley, chopped
6 tsp parmesan cheese, grated
8 cups broth
2 tbsp EVOO
Salt and pepper to taste

Instructions

- On a low heat, warm the oil in a large pan and sauté the onions until soft. Add garlic and red pepper flakes, and stir for 1 min. Increase to a medium heat and add the spinach and rice stir and cook for 2 mins. Pour in the broth. Simmer for 15 mins, until rice is soft. Remove from heat.
- In a small bowl, whisk eggs and lemon juice until a creamy consistency. Add a ladle of warmed (not hot) soup to the eggs and whisk. Slowly add another couple of ladles, to make sure the eggs do not curdle. Once it's not going to curdle, add the egg mixture to the soup. Stir and return to low heat. Heat through before serving.
- Garnish with parsley and grated parmesan.

Veggie Burgers

Serves: 6

Preparation Time: 15 minutes

Ingredients

1 large eggplant, sliced into rounds
6 oz haloumi cheese, sliced to roughly same size as eggplant
6 whole-wheat bread buns
2 tbsp extra virgin olive oil
Salt and pepper to season

Instructions

- Make pesto (ch 6)
- Heat 1 tbsp of oil in a skillet and sauté the eggplant, as you cook for 4 mins on each side. Sprinkle with salt and pepper, and set aside when cooked.
- Heat another 1 tbsp of oil in the skillet and add the cheese. Cook each side for 1-2 mins. Set aside when done.
- Open the burger buns and place on one side: a dollop of pesto, eggplant and halloumi. Place the other half of the bun on top and serve immediately.

Bean Salad

Serves: 2

Preparation Time: 15 minutes

Ingredients

1 1/2 cups tinned (or cooked) cannelloni beans
3 tbsp red onion, chopped
1/2 cup fresh parsley, chopped
1 tsp Dijon mustard
2 tbsp red wine vinegar
1/4 cup extra virgin olive oil
Salt and pepper to taste

Instructions

- Soak onions in cold water for 10 mins. Whisk mustard, vinegar and oil in a small bowl. Drain onions and add to the vinegar mix. Add beans, parsley, salt and pepper.
- Leave in fridge for 20 mins to allow the dressing to soak into the bean mix.

Stuffed Vine Leaves

Preparation Time: 60 minutes

Servings 5
Ingredients

1 x 15oz jar grape leaves, drained
1 x 19oz can chickpeas, washed and drained
1 cup cooked bulgur wheat
1 white onion, chopped fine
7 cloves garlic, minced
1 lemon zest and 1/2 cup lemon juice
3 tbsp tahini
1/2 cup fresh parsley leaves, chopped
2 tbsp extra virgin olive oil
Salt and pepper to taste

For serving
Lemon wedges
Bowl plain Greek yogurt

Instructions

- Boil water in a pot then turn down to medium heat, allowing it to simmer. Unravel grape leave and carefully place whole ones in the water to cook. Keep the broken leaves for another use. After 5 mins remove from the water and drain.
- Mix chickpeas with an electric mixer, until a rough consistency, set aside.
- In a food processor, combine the lemon zest and juice, garlic, tahini, salt and pepper, and mix until a smooth paste. Add the chickpeas, bulgur, parsley, and onions to the lemon paste.
- Flatten the grape leaves and add about 1-2 tsp of chickpea mixture. Fold the ends of leaves inside before rolling, so the rectangular shape is obtained.
- Place half of the broken grape leaves to cover the bottom of a large saucepan. Tuck as many of the stuffed grape leaf parcels on top as will fit. Drizzle with 2 tbsp lemon juice. Repeat a second layer of broken leaves and stuffed leaves on top, and again drizzle with lemon. Place a heatproof plate on top of the stuffed grape leaves. Put a heatproof bowl filled 3/4 with

water on top of that. This Serves as a weight. Now, pour water into the pan until it reaches the plate. The leaf parcels should be submerged. Bring water to boil, and then simmer for 30 mins.

- Serve warm on a platter with lemon wedges and a bowl of yogurt for dipping.
- Freeze or keep in airtight container for 3 days. Reheat in hot water.

Nutritional Value per serving: 38 calories, 1g fat(0 g sat), 2g fiber, 6g carbs; 1g protein.

Cod and Shrimp Soup

Servings 4

Preparation Time: 50 minutes

Ingredients

8oz cod fillets, chopped into 1 1/2 inch chunks
6oz shrimp peeled, deveined and slit lengthways
14 oz tomatoes, diced
10 oz can tomato puree
1 white onion, chopped
2 stalks celery, sliced
1 clove garlic, minced
1 tsp dried oregano
1 cup chicken broth
1/4 cup fresh parsley, chopped
1/4 cup dry white wine
1 tbsp extra virgin olive oil
Salt and pepper to taste
For serving
Lemon wedges
Bowl plain Greek yogurt
Instructions
- In a large pan heat the oil and sauté the onion and celery for 2 mins. Add garlic and cook another 1 min. Dispense the broth and wine. Bring to a boil, and then simmer for 5 mins. Add tomatoes, tomato puree, oregano, salt and pepper. Bring back to a boil, and then decrease to a simmer. Cover and cook for 5 mins.
- Bring back to a boil, then turn down to simmer for another 5 mins, adding all the fish.
- Once cooked, flake the fish with a fork and serve sprinkled with parsley.

Nutritional Value per serving: 165 calories, 4g fat (of which 1g sat), 2g fiber, 12g carbs, 19g protein.

Humble Oatmeal

Servings 1

Preparation Time: 20 minutes

Ingredients

1/2 cup oatmeal
1/4 cup olives of choice, pitted and halved
1/4 cup sun dried tomatoes, chopped
1/4 cup feta cheese, crumbled
1 clove garlic, minced
1/2 tsp dried oregano
1 cup vegetable broth
1 tbsp extra virgin olive oil
Salt and pepper to taste

Instructions

- Pour broth into a large pan, and bring to boil. Add oatmeal, oregano, salt and pepper. Simmer for 5 mins, stirring occasionally.
- In a skillet, heat 1/2 tbsp of oil and sauté the garlic, olives and tomatoes for 3 mins.
- Place oatmeal mixture in a small bowl and top with olive mixture. Sprinkle on feta and drizzle 1/2 tbsp oil over the top.
- Serve immediately.

Red Pepper Pasta

Servings 6

Preparation Time: 20 minutes

Ingredients

16 oz whole-wheat pasta, shape of choice
2 oz olives of choice, pitted and chopped
8 oz tomatoes, chopped
8 oz red bell pepper, diced
8 oz carrot, grated
2 oz white onions, chopped fine
1/4 cup plain Greek yogurt
1/4 cup mayonnaise
1 tbsp red wine vinegar
1 clove garlic, minced
1/2 tsp dried basil
2 tbsp extra virgin olive oil
Salt and pepper to taste

Instructions

Cook pasta as per packet **Instructions**.

Whisk together yogurt and mayonnaise. Add oil, vinegar, garlic, salt and pepper. Pour yogurt mixture over cooked pasta and stir. Add ALL uncooked and prepared vegetables, and toss.

May be served with warm or cold pasta.

Nutritional Value per serving: 215 calories, 9g fat (of which 1g sat), 4g fiber, 30g carbs, 6g protein.

Chapter 5: Flavored Mediterranean Diet Dinners

Cannelloni Beans Whole-wheat Stew

Serves: 6
Preparation Time: 30 minutes
Ingredients

2 carrots, diced small
2 sticks celery, cut into slices
1 onion, chopped
4 cups kale, chopped
15oz can cannelloni beans, drained and rinsed
15oz can chopped tomatoes
1 red bell pepper, roughly chopped into chunks
2 tbsp tomato paste
3 cloves garlic, minced

1 cup whole-wheat farro
1 tsp dried oregano
1tsp paprika
2 bay leaves
1/2 cup fresh parsley (keep whole with the stems)
1 tbsp lemon juice
5 cups vegetable broth
Salt and pepper to taste
4oz feta cheese, small crumbles

Instructions

- Heat the oil in a large pot,. Add carrots, celery, onions and sauté for 3 mins. Add the garlic and tomato paste. Pour the broth and tomatoes. Insert the peppers, farro, oregano, paprika, bay leaves, salt and pepper, and stir well. Bring to a boil and lay the parsley stems on top. Once boiling, turn down the heat and simmer for 15 mins.
- Remove pot from the heat and discard the parsley sprigs. Stir in the kale. Return to the heat and simmer for another 15 mins. Remove from heat once the farro is cooked through and add cannelloni beans. Let stand as the beans warm through and the farro swells. Add more hot water if consistency is too thick.
- Remove bay leaves and add lemon juice before serving. Sprinkle feta over the top.

Nutritional Value per serving: Calories 275, Carbs 46g, Fats 9g, Fiber 10g, Protein 15g

Chicken and Prunes with Rice

Serves: 4
Ingredients
Preparation Time: 25 minutes
Chicken legs and thighs - 8 pieces in all
1/2 cup of pitted prunes
1 tbsp capers
1 carrot, small cubes
1 white onion, finely chopped
1.3 cup pitted green olives
1/4 cup fresh flat leaf parsley, roughly chopped
3 clove garlic, minced
1 tsp dried oregano
1/3 cup white wine
3 tbsp red wine vinegar
1 tbsp brown sugar
Salt and pepper to taste
1 cup long grain rice (wild or brown is best)

Instructions
- Add white wine, vinegar, sugar, oregano, salt and pepper to a crock-pot and stir well. Add garlic, capers, prunes, olives. Lay the chicken pieces on top of the mixture. Cover and cook on Low for 5-6 hrs, OR High for 3-4 hrs.
- Stir the parsley around half hour before serving. At the same time, cook the rice according to packet Instructions.
- Serve by placing the chicken on top of the rice and pour the sauce over it all.

Salmon and Beet with Rice

Serves: 4
Ingredients
Preparation Time: 30 minutes
1lb salmon fillet slices (4 pieces)
2 medium golden beets, chopped into 1/2 inch chunks
8oz Brussel sprouts, halved
1 cup wild rice
1 carrot cut into small cubes
1 white onion, diced
1 lemon
2 tsp garlic, minced
1/2 tsp dried rosemary
1/2 tsp dried basil
1 tbsp pistachios, chopped
1/4 cup fresh flat leaf parsley, chopped
2 tbsp EVOO
Salt and pepper to taste

Instructions

- Set oven to 420F.
- Cook the rice as per the Instructions on the packet.
- In a bowl, add 1tbs oil with beets, sprouts salt and pepper. Place on a baking sheet and roast for 10 mins.
- Slice half the lemon. Add salmon to the vegetable baking tray, sprinkle with rosemary, salt and pepper, top with slices of lemon. Arrange vegetables to one side, salmon to other. Roast for up to 10 mins.
- Squeeze other half lemon for juice into a small bowl. Add garlic, the rest of the oil, basil, salt and pepper. Whisk.
- Serve with cooked rice, topped with roasted vegetables. Sit the salmon on top. Drizzle with lemon juice oil and sprinkle with pistachios.

Nutritional Value per serving: Calories 445. Carbs 45g, Fats - unsat 13g, sat 3g, Fiber 7g, Protein 32g

Harissa Baked Cod and Bulgur wheat

Serves: 2-3
Preparation Time: 25 minutes
Ingredients
2 large pieces of cod fillet
6oz cauliflower florets (not large stems)
2 large tomatoes, quartered
1 yellow pepper, chopped into large chunks
3 green onions, sliced
1 Lemon
2 oz bulgur wheat
2 tbsp Greek yoghurt
2 tsp Harissa paste
1 tsp dried cilantro
1 tsp extra virgin olive oil
Salt and pepper to taste
Instructions
- Preheat oven to 400F
- In a skillet, heat 1 tbsp oil. Add cauliflower, yellow peppers and sauté for 2 mins. Place on a baking tray with tomatoes and mix. Roast for 15 minutes.
- Boil 250ml of water in a small pan, then take off heat and add the bulgur wheat. Simmer for 2 mins then let stand.
- Cut the lemon in half. Squeeze the juice from one half, and thinly slice the other half.
- Remove vegetables from the oven and add the bulgur wheat, green onions, cilantro, salt and pepper. Drizzle the lemon juice, reserving a little. Coat the fish with Harissa paste and place on top of the bulgur mixture. Bake until the fish is cooked through, and then trickle the remaining lemon juice over it.
- Serve with Greek yoghurt on the side.

Nutritional value per serving: calories 453, protein 47g, 40g carbs 40g, fat 10g (of which 1g sat), fiber 9g.

Red Pepper Chicken and Quinoa

Serves: 4
Preparation Time: 20 minutes
Ingredients
1lb chicken breast, skinned and boneless
2 cups cooked quinoa
7oz jar roasted peppers
1/2 cup red onions, finely chopped
1 cup cucumber, diced into small chunks
1/4 cup chopped olives1/4 cup feta cheese, crumbled
1/4 cup sliced almond nuts
1 tsp pre-minced cooked garlic
1 tsp paprika
1/2 tsp ground cumin
2 tbsp fresh parsley, finely chopped
2 tbsp extra virgin olive oil
Salt and pepper to taste
Instructions

- Set the oven to 420F.
- Lay the chicken pieces on a lined baking tray and sprinkle with salt and pepper. Broil for 8 minutes, then turn the tray around and repeat.
- Add roasted peppers, almonds, garlic, paprika, cumin and 1 tbsp of the oil in a food processor and puree.
- Mix the cooked quinoa, onions, olives and 1 tbsp oil in a bowl.
- Divide the quinoa mixture evenly among the 4 bowls, and top with cucumber. Add chicken, then the roasted pepper puree. Garnish with parsley and crumbled feta.

Nutritional values per serving: 520 kcal, 32g protein, 30g carbs, 20g fat (of which 5g sat), 4g fiber.

Stuffed Pepper and Quinoa

Serves: 4

Preparation Time: 30 minutes

Ingredients

4 red bell peppers, halved and deseeded
1/2 cup white onions, finely chopped
1 zucchini, sliced
1/4 cup pitted and chopped olives
3 oz feta cheese, crumbled
16 oz quinoa, cooked
2 tbsp fresh parsley, finely chopped
2 tbsp extra virgin olive oil
Salt and pepper to taste

Instructions

- Heat oven to 350F
- Set the halved peppers, inside upwards, on a baking sheet. Add salt and pepper and drizzle with 1 tbsp oil. Bake for 15 mins.
- Heat up 1 tbsp oil in a skillet, and add the onions and zucchini. Once the onions are soft, remove pan from heat and add the cooked quinoa, olives, feta, parsley, salt and pepper.
- Divide the quinoa mixture between the halved peppers. Return to the oven and bake for a further 5 mins.
- Serve with a salad.

Roasted Lamb and Vegetables

Serves: 4

Preparation Time: 45 minutes

Ingredients

8 lamb cutlets, lean.
1 red onion, peeled, and quartered
1 large sweet potato, cut into medium chunks
2 bell peppers, cut into large chunks
2 zucchinis, sliced into 1inch chunks
1 tbsp dried thyme
1 tbsp dried mint
2 tbsp extra virgin olive oil
Salt and pepper to taste

Instructions

- Turn on the oven to 390F.
- Heat the oil in a skillet and sauté the sweet potato for 2 mins. Add red onions, pepper, zucchini, and sauté for 2 more mins. Pour contents onto a large flat baking tray. Season with salt and pepper. Cook for 5 mins. Remove from the oven and move the vegetable mix to one side of the tray.
- Trim any excess fat from the lamb. Sprinkle with thyme, mint, salt and pepper. Place lamb at the other side of the tray and return to the oven for another 10 mins. Take out and flip the lamb over. Put back in the oven for another 10 mins. Baste the mixed juices on the tray over the servings.

Nutritional value per serving: calories 430, protein 19g, carbs 23g, fat 29g, fibre 6g

Potato and Zucchini Bake

Serves: 4
Preparation Time: 20 minutes
Ingredients
2lb potatoes peeled, and sliced 1/8 inch thick
3 large zucchinis. sliced 1/8 inch thick
4 small onions, sliced 1/8 inch thick
4 tbsp tomato paste
1/2 cup water
4 tbsp extra virgin olive oil
Salt and Pepper to taste
Instructions
- Preheat oven to 400F
- Grease an ovenproof dish of at least 12x8x3 inches in size. Place the potatoes, onions and zucchini into the dish and mix. Add water to tomato puree and stir until blended, then poor over the potato mix. Add olive oil to the dish and stir. Season with salt and pepper. Bake for approx. 1h 30 mins, checking the progress every 30mins. Add a little more water if too dry..

Egg Plant Rolls

Serves: 2-3
Preparation Time: 35 minutes
Ingredients
1 large egg plant
1 white onion, sliced
1 cup mozzarella, cubed
1 red bell pepper, thinly sliced 1 zucchini, thickly sliced
6 tomatoes, roughly chopped
7 oz tomato paste
8 green olives, pitted
2 garlic cloves, minced
1/4 cup fresh basil, chopped
1 tbsp extra virgin olive oil
Salt and pepper to taste
Instructions
- Turn on oven to 350F
- Cut off the skin of the eggplant, and finely dice it. Slice the eggplant lengthways into long strips of approx.1/8in thick. Brush the slices with 1/2 tbsp of olive oil and fry on a griddle for 2-3 mins each side, or until tender. Take out of pan and set aside.
- Using the same pan, add the remaining oil and fry the diced eggplant, onions, half the garlic, red peppers, and sliced zucchini, until softened. Add the paste, salt and pepper to taste, and bring to the boil. Cook for 10 mins.
- In a bowl, combine tomatoes, olives, basil, mozzarella and remaining garlic. Spread out the slices of eggplant, and evenly divide the cooked paste mix at one end. Roll up the stuffed slices.
- Set them in an ovenproof dish, and pour over the tomato and mozzarella mix. Bake until the cheese melts. Serve while still hot.

Chicken Bake

Serves: 4
Preparation Time: 20 minutes
Ingredients
4 chicken breasts, skin included
2 red bell peppers, cut into large chunks
1 red onions, peeled and quartered
6oz cherry tomatoes
5 black olives, pitted
3oz garlic and herb soft cheese
1 tbsp dried tarragon
2 tsp extra virgin olive oil
Salt and pepper to taste
Instructions
Set the oven to 390F.
In a skillet Heat 1 tsp of oil. Add peppers, onions and sauté for 2 mins, ensure oil coats all the peppers and onion pieces. Place them onto a large baking tray. Cook in oven for 10 mins.
Lift the skin a little off the breast and push soft cheese underneath. Brush top of skin with remaining 1 tsp of oil. Sprinkle tarragon over skin. Remove the onions and peppers from oven. Add tomatoes and olives to onion and peppers. Scoot the vegetables to one side of baking tray. Place the chicken on the other side, leaving a gap between them and the veggie mix. Return to oven and for another 25 mins. Let the juices mix. Be sure that the chicken cooks thoroughly.
Nutritional value per serving: calories 400, protein 45g, carbs 9g, fat 21g, fiber 3g

Roasted Red Mullet Tomato salad

Serves: 2
Preparation Time: 20 minutes
Ingredients
2 red mullets
1/2 orange, juiced
1/2 lemon, juiced
1 tbsp chopped thyme
1 garlic clove, minced
Salad
6 oz plum tomatoes
2 oz thinly sliced Fennel
1 tsp lemon juice
4 oz broad beans
2 oz olives, pitted
5 mint leaves finely chopped
1 tsp sea salt
Dressing
1 tsp fresh oregano, chopped
1 tbsp extra virgin olive oil
Lemon juice to taste
Instructions
- Heat oven to 425F
- Cut two slashes on each side of the fish.
- Whisk together the lemon juice, orange juice, chopped thyme and garlic. Pour over mullets, turning the fish to ensure it's completely covered. Place in an ovenproof dish, and cook for 12 mins, or until cooked through.
- Combine ALL salad **Ingredients** and sprinkle with sea salt. Put in fridge for 5 mins.
- Combine ALL dressing **Ingredients** in a jar with a lid and shake until emulsified. Pour dressing over the salad, and toss until coated.
- Serve with a salad by its side.

Ras-el-hanout baked chicken

Serves: 4
Preparation Time: 20 minutes
Ingredients
4 chicken breasts, boned and skinned
1lb sweet potatoes, peeled and cubed
1lb cubed carrots
1 large red onion, peeled and cut into wedges
3 whole garlic cloves
1 lemon, quartered
4 tbsp Greek yogurt
2 tsp ras-el-hanout
1 tsp dried cilantro leaf
1 tsp dried thyme
1 tbsp extra virgin olive oil
Salt and pepper to taste
Instructions
- Preheat oven to 400F.
- Place carrots and sweet potatoes on a baking tray. Drizzle with the olive oil, bake for 10 minutes. Remove from oven and add red onion and garlic. Bake for 20 mins more.
- Move the vegetables to one side of the tray and place the chicken breasts and lemon quarters. Bake until the chicken cooks through. Allow the juices to blend.
- Split between four bowls and serve with a tbsp of yogurt on top.

Nutritional Values per serving: 361 kcal, 44g protein, 30g carbs, 5.5g fat (of which 1g sat), 7g fiber.

Cinnamon Chicken and Chickpeas

Serves: 4

Preparation Time: 30 minutes
(Not including making couscous - see the recipe for the timing)

Ingredients

1 whole rotisserie chicken, skinned and deboned, cut into bite size pieces
15oz can chickpeas, drained and rinsed
28 oz can tomatoes, diced
1 red bell pepper, cut into large chunks
1 small carrot, shredded
1 onion, finely chopped
1 garlic clove, minced
1/2 cup olives, pitted and chopped
1 tsp dried oregano
1 tsp dried parsley
2 bay leaves
1 cup chicken broth
1 tbsp lemon juice
2 tbsp extra virgin olive oil
Salt and pepper to taste
Cinnamon couscous (see recipe chapter 6)

Instructions

- Heat oven to 390 F.
- In a skillet with heated oil, add the onions and carrots and sauté for 2 mins until soft. Add peppers, garlic, oregano, parsley and sauté for another 2 minutes. Pour in the tomatoes, chick peas, olives, broth, bay leaves, salt and pepper. Bring to a boil then simmer for 5 mins. Add the chicken and simmer uncovered, for 10 more mins to heat through the meat. Remove from heat. Discard the bay leaves, add olives and lemon juice.
- Meanwhile, cook the cinnamon couscous as per our recipe in chapter 6.
- Serve on a bed of couscous.

Beef Meat balls Greek Style

Serves: 5

Preparation Time: 30 minutes

Ingredients
Meatballs:

1lb lean ground beef
5 whole wheat pita breads
1/2 red onion, chopped
1 tbsp dried ginger
2 cloves garlic, grated
1 tsp dried parsley
1/2 tsp dried mint
1 tbsp ground coriander
1/2 tsp ground cloves
1 tbsp cumin
1/2 tsp cinnamon
1/2 tsp red pepper flakes
2 tbsp extra virgin olive oil
salt and pepper to taste
Yogurt dip (Tzatziki)
1 whole cucumber
1/2 onion, grated
2 lemons, zested and juiced
1 cup plain Greek yogurt
1 garlic clove, grated fine
1/2 cup fresh dill, finely chopped
1 tsp dried mint (or 1/2 cup fresh chopped)
2 tbsp extra virgin olive oil
salt and pepper to taste
Instructions
- Make the Tzatziki first, as it needs to marinade:

- Cut 1/4 of the cucumber, and dice into cubes. Peel and grate the remaining 3/4 of cucumber. Place the grated cucumber in a small bowl and sprinkle with salt. Set aside for 15 mins.
- In another bowl, combine 1 tbsp lemon peel, 2 tbsp lemon juice, garlic, dill, mint and oil. Season with salt and pepper.
- Wring out the excess liquid from the grated cucumber; either with your hands, or place the grated cucumber in a sieve and press with the back of a spoon. Add it to the lemon mix. Chill in the fridge for at least 1 hr.
- To make the meatballs:
- In a separate bowl, combine the onions, ginger, garlic, parsley, mint, ground beef, coriander, cloves, cumin, and cinnamon. Season with salt and pepper. Mix well but be careful not to overwork it. The less handling it gets- the better. Divide into 30 balls.
- Heat oil in a skillet on medium heat and fry meatballs a few at a time, until browned and cooked through. Place under a low grill as you cook them, to keep them warm.
- Sprinkle the pitas with water and warm them under the grill, or in an , careful not to brown them too much. Top them with meatballs and the Greek sauce. Garnish with red onion and diced cucumber.

Pasta and Eggplant

Serves: 4

Preparation Time: 15 minutes
Ingredients
8oz whole meal penne pasta
1 small eggplant, diced
2 garlic cloves, finely diced
1 red chili pepper, finely diced
14oz can tomatoes, diced
1 tsp dried basil
2 tbsp dried cheese, such as parmesan
2 tbsp extra virgin olive oil
Instructions
- Cook the pasta according to package Instructions.
- While pasta is cooking, heat 1 tbsp of oil in a skillet. Add eggplant in batches, until golden brown, and then set aside. In same pan, cook garlic and diced chili for 5 mins. Add tomatoes, bring to a boil, and then simmer for 10 mins. Stir the pasta in, and cook for a further 5 mins.
- Serve in bowls, sprinkled with dried cheese.

Chapter 6: Amazing Mediterranean Diet SNACKS

Pita Chips

Serves: 4   **Preparation Time:** 10 minutes
(Not including making pita breads - see our recipe for timings of this)
Ingredients
2 large whole-wheat pita breads (see our recipe in this chapter to make them)
2 Tbsp extra virgin olive oil

Instructions
Cut pita breads into 16 portions. Spread out on a baking sheet and brush with 2 tbsp olive oil. Bake at 350F, for approx 6 mins on each side. Use more oil if needed, to make sure every piece is covered.

Greek Nachos

Serves: 4   **Preparation Time:** 20 minutes
(Not including making pita chips or hummus - see our recipe for the timing)
Ingredients
3 cups pita chips (see our recipe in Snacks)
1/3 cup hummus (see our recipe in Snacks)
2 tbsp white onion, chopped
1/2 cup cherry tomatoes, quartered
1/4 cup feta cheese, crumbled
2 tbsp olives, sliced
1 cup lettuce, shredded
Pepper to taste
2 tbsp extra virgin olive oil
1 tbsp fresh oregano
1 tbsp lemon juice

Instructions
- Whisk together oil, lemon juice, oregano, pepper, and stir in the hummus.
- Spread pita chips over a large platter. Distribute most of the hummus on top, saving a little for later. Cover with lettuce, onions, tomatoes, olives, feta. Top with the rest of the hummus mixture.

Easy hummus

Serves: 4   **Preparation Time:** 5 minutes
Ingredients
2 garlic cloves, crushed   2 tbsp fresh lemon juice
7oz can chickpeas   4 tbsp water
1 tbsp Tahini   1 tbsp extra virgin olive oil
1 tsp Paprika   Salt to taste
1 tsp cumin
Instructions
Drain and rinse the chickpeas. In a blender or food processor, combine the olive oil, lemon juice, water, garlic, cumin and tahini, and blend until a smooth puree. Sprinkle with paprika and serve with warmed quartered pita breads.

Nutritional Value: per serving = Calories 160, Carbs 13g, Fats - unsat 8g, sat 2g, Fiber 2g, Protein 4g

Crunchy Chickpeas

Serves: 4   **Preparation Time:** 10 minutes
Ingredients
2 x 15 oz cans chickpeas, rinsed   1/2 tsp chili powder
and drained   1/2 tsp turmeric
1 tsp curry powder   2 tbsp EVOO
1 tsp cumin   Salt to taste
Instructions
- Make sure the chickpeas are completely dry and remove any loose skins. Put them in a bowl and add oil and salt, stirring to make sure all chickpeas are covered. Place in center of oven at 400F for 30 mins, turning over every 10 mins. Don't worry if they pop.
- Mix all spices and salt together.
- Immediately the chickpeas are crispy on the outside, take out of oven and sprinkle with the spice mix.
- Serve while warm otherwise, they lose their crispiness.

Greek Panzanella

Serves: 9 on a sharing platter
Ingredients
16 oz artisan bread loaf, torn into 1-inch pieces (10 cups)
6 oz feta cheese, crumbled
3lb tomatoes, roughly chopped 1 small red onion, thinly sliced
1 cup pitted olives

Preparation Time: 20 minutes

2 tbsp fresh oregano, roughly chopped
4 tbsp fresh lemon juice
3 tbsp extra virgin olive oil
Salt and pepper to taste

Instructions
- The day prior, spread the bread pieces on an oven tray, so it hardens overnight. OR bake at 300F for around 15 mins to crisp up.
- Soak the onion slices in a bowl of cold water for approximately 10 mins.
- In a separate large bowl add the tomatoes and olives and mix.
- To make the dressing for the salad, whisk the oil, lemon juice, oregano, salt and pepper in a jug.
- Drain the onions and add to the bowl with tomato and olive mix. Add the bread pieces and pour the marinade over. Mix well. Let stand for up to 4 hrs. Stir occasionally to ensure the lemon juice covers all the Ingredients.
- Mix in the feta before serving. Enjoy the same day.

Cinnamon Couscous

Serves: 4
Preparation Time: 5 minutes

Ingredients
10 oz whole-wheat couscous
1/3 cup raisins
2 tsp cinnamon
1 tsp dried cilantro

2 cups chicken broth
2 tbsp orange juice
1 tbsp extra virgin olive oil
Salt and pepper to taste

Instructions
Place the broth in a pan and bring to a boil. Add the oil, salt and pepper. Remove from the heat and add couscous, raisins and cilantro. Let stand for 5 mins. Add cinnamon and orange juice, fluffing the couscous with a fork.

Feta Dip

Servings 8
Preparation Time: 10 minutes
Ingredients

8 oz feta cheese, small crumbles
8 oz ricotta cheese
2 oz pre-cooked hot chili peppers

4 oz pre-roasted bell peppers, chopped
1 tsp cayenne pepper, or to taste
1 tsp lemon juice

Instructions
- Puree the chili, bell peppers and cayenne in a food processor, until a smooth paste. Add the crumbled feta and stir.
- In a separate bowl, combine the ricotta cheese and lemon juice. Add to the feta mix and stir until combined.
- Serve chilled.

Nutritional Values per serving: 134 calories, 9.3 g fat, 4.2 g carbohydrates, 8.3 g protein.

Halloumi Sticks

Servings 8
Preparation Time: 10 minutes
Ingredients

6 oz halloumi cheese, cut into sticks of 1/2-inch thickness, 3-4 inches long
1/4 tsp dried oregano
2 tsp lemon juice
1/2 tbsp extra virgin olive oil
Black pepper to taste

Instructions

Heat the oil in a skillet. Add cheese sticks and oregano, cooking either side for 1-2 mins. Place on a small plate and sprinkle with lemon juice and pepper.

Nutritional Values per serving: 299 calories, 24.7g fat, 3g carbs, 18g protein.

Feta Triangle

Servings 8
Preparation Time: 20 minutes
Ingredients

8 sheets filo pastry
6 oz feta cheese, crumbled
2 oz gouda cheese, grated
2 oz hard Italian cheese such as parmesan

1 egg
1/4 cup fresh dill, chopped
1 tbsp milk
1 tbsp extra virgin olive oil
Black pepper to taste

Instructions

- Heat oven to 320 F.
- Crush the feta cheese with the back of a spoon in a large bowl. Add the gouda, egg, milk, dill, and pepperMix well.
- Spread out 1 sheet of filo and brush with oil, lay another filo sheet on top, again brushing with oil. Cut the pastry sheets into 4. At one end of each cut, place 1 tbsp of cheese filling. Fold over the edges into a triangle. Repeat with remaining filo pastry sheets, until you have 8 stuffed triangles.
- Oil a baking tray and place the pastry triangles on it. Brush the tops with remaining oil. Use more oil if needed. Bake for 20-25 mins.
- Serve warm or cold.

Spicy Pesto

Serves: 2
Preparation Time: 5 minutes
Ingredients

3 tbsp shelled pistachios, toasted
1 small white onion, chopped
1 cup fresh cilantro
1 cup fresh parsley
1/2 cup fresh mint leaves

1 tsp chili flakes
1 lemon, zest and juice
1 tsp white wine vinegar
1 tbsp extra virgin olive oil
Salt and pepper to taste

Instructions

Combine ALL Ingredients in a food processor bowl and blend to your preferred consistency of pesto.

Pita Bread

Servings 6
Preparation Time: 15 minutes
Ingredients

2 cups all-purpose flour *(could use half wholewheat flour)*
1 tsp dry yeast

1 tsp salt
1 tsp sugar
Luke warm water as necessary

Instructions

- Sieve flour into your mixer bowl. Add yeast, sugar and salt. Add water gradually, as you start mixing and creating dough. Add more water if the dough is crumbly, if sticky; add more flour. Allow to sit in a warm place for 30 mins, or until doubled in size.
- Knead the dough, but only a little, then divide into 6 portions. Roll out or stretch until flat and 1 cm thick. With a fork, create a few holes on the surface.
- Dry fry each portion in a skillet on medium heat, for 3 mins each side.

Pita Pizza

Servings 8
Preparation Time: 15 minutes
(Not including making pitas or pesto - see our recipe for the timing)
Ingredients
4 pitas (see our recipe, in this chapter)
14 oz mozzarella cheese, grated
1 large tomato, sliced
4 tbsp tomato paste
1/2 tsp dried oregano
2 tsp pesto (see our recipe, in this chapter)
1 cup of green salad leaves
Salt and pepper to taste
Instructions
- Heat oven to 250 F.
- Place the pitas on flat baking tray, and spread 1 tbsp of tomato paste(per pita) on the top. Sprinkle with oregano, salt and pepper. Spread 1/2 tsp pesto over each pita. Sprinkle with mozzarella, add slices of tomato and sprinkle with more mozzarella. Bake in the oven for 10 mins, or until the cheese melts.
- Leave to cool a little, then cut each ptta in half. Serve with a small green salad.

Eggplant Crunchy Bites

Serves: 4

Preparation Time: 15 minutes

Ingredients

2 eggplants, sliced into rounds approx. 1/2 inch thick

350 ml light beer of choice

7 oz all-purpose flour

Extra light olive oil (or sunflower oil) for frying

Salt and pepper to taste

Instructions

- Spread out eggplant slices and sprinkle with table salt on both sides. Set aside on extra thick kitchen paper. This will help draw out the excess water. After 30 mins, brush salt off with a dry cloth and pat dry.
- Into a large bowl pour the beer and sift in the flour, stirring as you go, to avoid lumps. Add salt and pepper to taste. Batter should resemble thick cream in consistency, not be too thin and runny. Chill for 30 mins. Dip eggplant slices into the batter mix, making sure they are fully coated.
- In a skillet, heat the oil to a medium high heat and fry the eggplant in batter, for approximately 1-2mins. Make sure both sides are crispy. Place on dry cloth to remove excess oil.

Calamari Rings

Serves: 4

Preparation Time: 20 minutes

Ingredients

25 oz calamari, sliced 1/2 thick

3.5 oz bread flour

1.5 oz semolina flour

1/2 tbsp paprika

1/2 tbsp dried oregano

Extra light olive oil (or sunflower oil) for frying

Salt and pepper to taste

Instructions

- Wash calamari slices and pat dry with paper towels, or clean cloth.
- Add ALL flours, paprika, oregano, salt and pepper to a large bowl and mix. Rub each piece of the calamari in the flour mixture, making sure all sides are covered. Fry in a large pan with hot oil.
- Serve with a squeeze of lemon juice and a tasty dip.

Chapter 7: Great Mediterranean Diet Desserts

Greek Rice pudding

Serves: 6

Preparation Time: 5 minutes
Ingredients
4oz short grain rice, uncooked
2 pints whole milk
4 tbsp castor sugar
1 tsp vanilla extract
1/2 tsp ground cinnamon
Instructions
- Add rice and milk to pan, and bring to boil. Reduce to a simmer, stirring occasionally, until the milk is absorbed, approx. 35mins. The rice should have a creamy texture. Add sugar and vanilla extract, and stir until sugar dissolves. Add a little corn flour to thicken, if the rice mix is too thin and runny,. If too thick, add a little more milk and stir well.
- Dust with ground cinnamon. Serve hot or cold.

Raspberry Frozen Yogurt

Servings 15 scoops (approx.)

Preparation Time: 10 minutes
Ingredients
24 fl oz Greek yogurt
8 oz raspberries, chopped
8 oz icing sugar
2 tsp vanilla extract
Pinch of sea salt
3 tbsp lemon juice
Instructions
- Add ALL Ingredients into a bowl, and stir until smooth. Pour into a freezer safe lidded container and pop into a freezer. Remove every 30 mins and stir the mixture. Keep doing this until it freezes completely. This method helps stops ice crystals from forming.
- Let stand at room temperature for 5-10 mins before serving

Baklava

Serves: 2

Preparation Time: 20 minutes
Ingredients
10 sheets of readymade filo pastry
3 oz unsalted butter
4 oz mixed pistachios and walnuts, chopped
1 tbsp castor sugar
1/2 tsp ground cinnamon
Syrup
5 oz castor sugar
5 oz water
1 tbsp lime juice
1 tsp vanilla extract
Instructions
- Preheat the oven to 350 F.
- Melt the butter. Grease baking tray with melted butter and lay 5 sheets of the filo pastry on it, brushing each layer with melted butter.
- Combine sugar, nuts, and cinnamon in a bowl and mix. Spread nut mixture over the top sheet of filo pastry. Lay the remaining sheets of pastry on top of the nut mixture, again brushing each layer with a little butter.
- Cut a criss-cross pattern on the top layer. Bake for around 30-40 mins. Set aside to cool when done.

Syrup: Put the sugar, water, lemon juice and vanilla extract into a saucepan. Heat slowly until all sugar has dissolved, and created syrup. Once cooled, pour over the baklava. Cut into small diamond shaped pieces when completely cooled.

Halva

Serves: 4

Preparation Time: 10 minutes
Ingredients
1 cup uncooked semolina
1 cup sliced almonds
3 cups castor sugar
3 cinnamon sticks
1 tbsp ground cinnamon
3 cloves
1 cup honey
4 cups water
1 cup extra virgin olive oil
Instructions
- Add the water to a pan along with sugar, cinnamon sticks and cloves. Boil gently for 5 mins. Take Remove from heat and discard the cloves and cinnamon sticks. Add the honey and set aside.
- In a separate pan, heat the oil and add semolina, constantly stirring until the mixture turns a golden brown. Add 1/2 tsp of ground cinnamon. Slowly pour sugar syrup, onto the semolina mix. Keep the heat on, and keep stirring as it thickens. Add the almonds and continue to stir. When everything is combined, move the Halva mixture to a domed glass bowl and leave to cool. Flip onto a plate and sprinkle with remaining ground cinnamon.

Mediterranean Pancakes

Servings 4-6   **Preparation Time:** 5 minutes

Ingredients

16 oz all-purpose flour
1 tsp castor sugar
1/2 tsp cinnamon
1 tsp dried yeast
2 cups tepid water
2 tbsp extra virgin olive oil
pinch of salt

Instructions

- In a bowl combine the water and yeast, and stir until the yeast dissolves. Add flour, sugar, salt and cinnamon, and whisk into a smooth batter. Cover, and set aside for 10 -15 minutes until bubbles form on top of the batter.
- Heat 1 tbsp oil to large frying pan. Pour 1-2 tbsp of batter into the pan in separate blobs to cook 2-3 at a time. Repeat.
- Place on a paper towel to soak up excess oil. Serve warm with Greek yogurt, honey and chopped walnuts.

Bougatsa

Serves: 8-10

Preparation Time: 25 minutes
Ingredients
35 fl oz milk
Zest of 1 lemon
6 oz semolina
14 oz castor sugar
4 eggs (room temp)
1/4 tsp vanilla extract
12 sheets filo Pastry
4 oz unsalted butter, melted
Instructions
- In a bowl mix the eggs, lemon zest, sugar and vanilla, and whisk until foamy.
- Heat milk in a pan, but do not boil. Add the semolina to the warm milk and stir until mixture is smooth and thick. Stirring, slowly add the egg mixture. Remove from heat and pour into a glass bowl. Leave to cool for 5 mins, then cover the surface with cling wrap. Put it in thefridge to cool.
- Brush a baking tray that is slightly smaller than the unrolled filo with melted butter. Layer 8 sheets of filo, brushing each sheet with butter, and allowing the edges of the sheets to overlap the tin.
- Spread the now cooled custard filling over the filo sheets. Turn the overlapping edges inside, brushing them with melted butter. Place remaining filo sheets on top and again brush each sheet with melted butter.
- Bake at 350 F for 30-40 minutes, or until the top is a golden brown.
- Cool before cutting into slices.

Roasted Figs with Spicy Mascarpone

Serves: 4

Preparation Time: 10 minutes

Ingredients

8 figs, halved and trimmed
2 tbsp butter
2 tbsp clear honey
2 tbsp sugar
4 oz Mascarpone

1 piece of stem ginger, cut into small pieces
2 tsp ground cinnamon
1 tbsp ginger root syrup
2 tbsp pure orange juice

Instructions

- Heat oven to 400 F.
- Lay figs on a baking tray with a small blob of butter on each one. Drizzle with honey, sugar, orange juice and cinnamon.
- Bake for 15 minutes.
- Add syrup and ginger to the mascarpone and mix . Top each fig with the mascarpone mix, and serve warm.

Lemon muffins

Servings: 12
Preparation Time: 10 minutes
Ingredients
4 large free range eggs
3 fl oz low fat Greek yoghurt
1 tbsp lemon zest, grated fine
8oz all-purpose flour *(could replace half with whole-wheat)*
1 tbsp baking powder
7 oz castor sugar
4 fl oz extra virgin olive oil
Pinch of salt
Instructions
- Heat oven to 350 F.
- Sift flour, salt and baking powder into a large bowl.
- Combine eggs and sugar in a separate bowl, and whisk until mixture is pale and creamy. Add yogurt and olive oil, and continue whisking until blended. Add flour mix, and fold into the liquid stirring it in slowly. Divide the mixture into 12 greased muffin tins.
- Bake for 15 minutes. Cool for 5 mins in the baking tin when done, then flip them out of the tin, and finish cooling on a wire rack.

Greek Chocolate Yogurt Mousse

Serves: 4

Preparation Time: 10 minutes

Ingredients

7 oz milk chocolate

7 oz dark chocolate

2 digestive biscuits, crumbled

7 oz Greek yogurt, strained

1/5 cup warm milk

Instructions

- Break up both chocolates, and melt in the microwave or in a bowl over a pan of boiling water. Be careful not to get it too hot or it will burn. Add the lukewarm milk to the melted chocolate and stir until blended. Then combine the yogurt into the chocolate mix.
- Serve in glass dessert bowls with crushed digestive biscuits sprinkled on top.

Yogurt and Summer fruits

Serves: 6

Preparation Time: 10 minutes

Ingredients

8 oz of mixed raspberries and strawberries

2 fl oz sweet dessert wine

4 tbsp castor sugar (or sweetener)

8 fl oz cream

8 fl oz Greek yoghurt

Mint leaves as garnish

Instructions

- In a bowl add the fruit and sprinkle with sugar. Let it sit for 5-10 minutes. Whip the cream until soft peaks form, and then stir in the yogurt. Add the fruit to the yogurt mixture, and stir until you have a rippled effect.
- Serve in dessert glasses topped with a mint leaf.

Mediterranean Honey Cake

Serves: 12

Preparation Time: 20 minutes

Ingredients

1 cup all-purpose flour *(could replace half with whole-wheat)*
1 1/2 tsp baking powder
3/4 cup butter
1 3/4 cup white sugar
3 eggs
1/4 cup milk
1 cup walnuts, chopped fine
1 cup honey
Zest of 1 orange
1/2 tsp ground cinnamon
3/4 cup water
1 tsp lemon juice freshly squeezed
Pinch of salt

Instructions

- Heat oven to 350F
- In a bowl, add the flour, baking powder, and salt, cinnamon and orange zest. Stir until combined.
- In a separate bowl, add the butter, 3/4 cup of sugar, and cream until light and fluffy. Whisk in the eggs, one at a time until combined. Add the flour mix and beat until smooth. Add some milk if too thick. Insert the walnuts to the mixture. Pour the cake mix into a square 9in greased cake tin, and bake for 40 mins.
- Insert a thin knife blade to see if it's cooked. If it comes out clean, it's done. Remove from oven and cool on a wire rack.
- For the syrup, combine honey, lemon juice, remaining sugar and water in a small saucepan. Bring to a simmer for 6 mins.
- Cut into even squares and pour syrup evenly over the cake before serving.

Greek Parfait

Serves: 2

Preparation Time: 10 minutes

Ingredients

12 fl oz Greek yogurt
1 mango, pitted, cut into small cubes

2-3 oz chopped pistachios
2-3 oz pomegranate seeds
1 tsp squeezed orange juice

Instructions

- Stir orange juice into yogurt.
- Divide mango between two dessert bowls. Cover the fruit with a layer of yogurt mix. Sprinkle with pistachios. Cover nuts with remaining yogurt, and garnish with pomegranate seeds.
- Chill in the refrigerator until ready to serve.

Bottomless Cheesecake

Serves: 6

Preparation Time: 15 minutes

Ingredients

32 oz ricotta cheese
6 eggs
5 oz sugar
2 oz all-purpose flour

1/4 tsp ground cinnamon
2 tsp orange zest
1 tsp vanilla extract

Instructions

- Heat oven to 300F
- Put the Ricotta into a bowl, and beat until smooth. Add sugar and flour and mix together. Add one egg at a time, mixing each one into the cheese mixture. Stir in the orange zest, cinnamon and vanilla extract. Pour into a greased 9in spring-form cake tin and bake for 90 minutes.
- Cool on a wire rack, Let it stand for 10 mins before removing from tin..
- Serve Chilled.

Nut stuffed Baked figs

Servings 12

Preparation Time: 15 minutes
Ingredients
12 Dried whole figs
6 oz walnuts, finely chopped
1 tbsp cocoa powder
Pinch of ground cinnamon
2 tbsp honey
2 tbsp cranberry juice
1 tsp lemon juice
Instructions
- Heat oven to 350 F.
- Remove the fig stems, and cut an X in the top, about 3/4 of the way down.
- Combine the walnuts, 1 tbsp of honey, cocoa and cinnamon in a bowl, and stir until all nuts are well coated. Stuff the figs with nut mixture.
- Combine lemon juice, cranberry juice and remaining honey in a jug. Whisk until blended and pour over the figs.
- Cover with foil and bake for 20 mins. Uncover and bake for another 10 mins.
- Serve warm with a little mascarpone or fresh cream.

Nutritional Values per serving: 98 calories, 3g fat (0 sat), 14g carbs, Fiber 3g,1g protein.

Baked Honey Pecan Pears

Serves: 4
Preparation Time: 5 minutes
Ingredients
2 large pears, cut in half (ripe ones are best for this recipe)
2 tsp honey
2 oz pecans chopped fine
Instructions
- Set oven to 350F
- Lay the pears on a baking tray, with the cut side up. Sprinkle pears with pecans and drizzle with honey.
- Bake for 30 minutes.
- Cool slightly before eating. Serve with Greek yogurt.

Nutritional Values per serving: 111 calories, 5g fat (0 sat), 17g carbs, Fiber 3g,1.5g protein.

The Final Words

This is only the beginning, if you have decided to join the growing popularity of the Mediterranean style diet. Within these pages, you have found many delicious recipes, but these are only to get you started. Once you completed the 2-week menu plan, you will have a fine idea of the types of food to include in your future meal planning. The recipes are infinite. It's all about cutting out the unhealthy foods. You too will see that are plenty of nutritious and delicious Ingredients available to make healthy and tasty meals.

Many studies looked at the Mediterranean lifestyle. It's because the natives of these regions live longer and healthier lives. That is enough to make you wonder how they do it. Plenty of sunshine is, of course, a great advantage. Though it is that hot sun that leads to lack of cattle in the Mediterranean. Less meat and more fruits, vegetables, and seafood. This proves we don't need to consume lots of meat in our diet. We can lead a healthier life by eating a lot of vegetables and fruit, just as the natives of the Mediterranean.

By adding oily fish to your diet, you fulfill all the requirements the Mediterranean diet recommends. Eating these healthy Ingredients, and cutting out refined processed foods will help you lose excess weight. No need to go hungry; just watch portion sizes and, for the sake of your heart, include exercise in your daily regime.

Try to reach the following lists of food, if possible:

DAILY
- 3tbs olive oil.
- 6 portions of vegetables.
- 1 handful of nuts.
- 3 servings of fruit.

WEEKLY
- 3 servings of legumes.
- 2 meals of fish.
- 4 servings of a few eggs.
- 2 dairy in the form of cheese or yogurt.
- 6 meals with whole grains.

Made in the USA
Middletown, DE
18 April 2019